TRICKS

OF

TRADE

IN

NEUROLOGY

DR. IFTIKHAR KHAWAJA

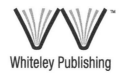

Whiteley Publishing

Published by Whiteley Publishing Ltd
www.whiteleypublishing.com
First paperback edition 2015
Illustration by: Mohammad Ali Talpur
ISBN 978-1-908586-59-9

"The Neurological Examination of an unconscious patient is the most dreaded of all. Examination of an acutely confused neurological patient without appropriate skills is like searching for a black cat in a dark room.

Tricks of the Trade is well presented, easy to understand and enjoyable. This guide is surely to become part of junior doctor's essential tools to survive foundation year training.

The stroke team of Great Western Hospital, Swindon are very grateful for this wonderful gift to the department!"

Dr. Shivprasad Siddegowda
Consultant Stroke Physician

Foreword

According to the Royal College of Physicians of London, learning to make a difference is all about empowering junior doctors to learn and develop skills in quality improvement and put those new skills into practice to make a real difference to their patient care.

This book is meant to inspire junior doctors to improve their own learning and skills in Neurology through an easy to follow introduction to the subject.

A trick of the trade is what the professionals automatically do. Although it does not replace a proper grounding in the discipline, this little book will help improve the trainee doctors' ability to examine neurological patients, and understand what they are doing, from the very first day of induction.

Dr. Iftikhar Khawaja

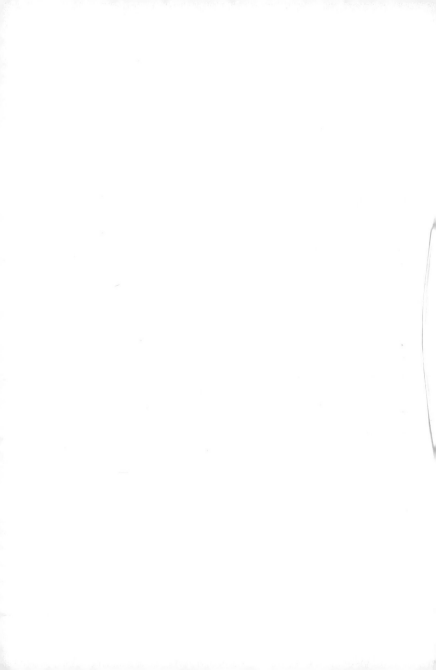

Acknowledgements

Special thanks are due to Dr. Merek Kunc, Consultant Neurologist, Airedale Hospital, Yorkshire, for revising the book, pointing out some ambiguities and providing helpful suggestions. Thanks are due to Shirley Elkins and Pamela Quesnel for typing and arranging the original text. Thanks are also due to Donna Hill for painstakingly organising the revised text and putting it in a printable format.

Special thanks are due to Mohammad Ali Talpur for taking time to beautifully illustrate the text. Thanks are also due to my sons Edward and Nik for their encouragement and technical support.

Lastly thanks are due to all the junior doctors who read and used these little "tricks" in the wards as a practical demonstration to prove that they do work!

Introduction

Neurology is a subject that needs to be taught with passion. Neurological examination is a form of art that can be mastered by learning from good clinicians.

Dr. Khawaja is an excellent clinical neurologist who is eager to disseminate his knowledge amongst junior doctors.

This book is not intended to replace well known text books in neurology but it is a collection of practical easy snippets for junior doctors to remember and practise.

I am extremely grateful to Dr. Khawaja for sharing this book with my junior doctors.

Dr. Sunil Punnoose
Consultant Stroke Physician
Rotherham General Hospital

What Is Common Between Central Nervous System And Domestic Power Supply?

The Central Nervous System (CNS) is like the main box in a power supply from which cables arise to connect to various electrical appliances like kettle, toaster, iron etc.

The first part, including the big box and the major cables are the upper motor neurons in the CNS, which include cerebral cortex and corticospinal fibres.

The appliances and the electric connections including sockets are the lower motor neurons, which include anterior horn cells, nerve roots, peripheral nerves and muscles.

How To Assess Whether An Unconscious Patient Has Had A Stroke Or Not

"Patient was unconscious. Therefore a neurological examination was not possible." (from A&E notes)

What are your bedside observations?

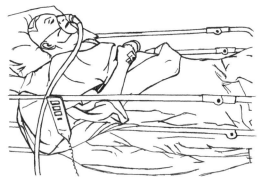

In an unconscious patient with suspected stroke.

Observation 1 - Head and eyes turned to one side

A. If you can't work out why it happens, remember the normal hemisphere pushes the head and eyes to the opposite side.

Thus if head and eyes are turned to the left, it means the right hemisphere is doing the pushing, which means the left hemisphere is

not working.

Result: Right hemiparesis.

Observation 2

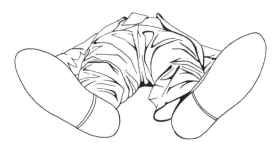

Paralysed limb flops when you lift it and let it drop.

Observation 3

Paralysed limb fails to move when noxious stimulus is applied, while the normal limb moves in response to the noxious stimulus. Therefore the normal limb will move (unless GCS is low) but paralysed limb will remain immobile.

3

Muscle Tone

If a guitar string is loose, it has low tone. The more you tighten it, the higher the tone is.

Think upper motor neuron if the tone is high. Upper for Higher.

High / Low formula:

Higher note in the guitar string = **Higher Tone**
Higher tone means **Upper Motor** Neuron

Lower note in the guitar string = **Lower Tone**
Lower tone means **Lower Motor** Neuron

How to test the tone

On passive movement of a joint, for instance ankle, with low tone, you will find the joint rather floppy. Conversely, if you meet with undue resistance while moving the joint passively, the tone is high.

Golden Rule:

Low tone = LMN High tone = UMN

4

Muscle Power

How to test

Always use your strongest muscle groups and apply resistance after explaining to the patient what you want him/her to do.

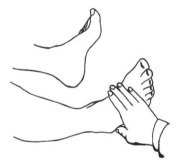

Figure 1. Testing dorsiflexion.

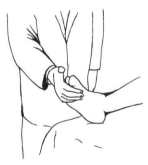

Figure 2. Testing plantar flexion.

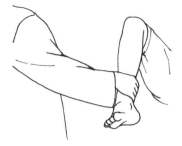

Figure 3. Testing knee flexion.

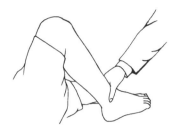

Figure 4. Testing knee extension.

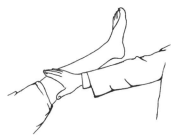

Figure 5. Testing hip flexion.

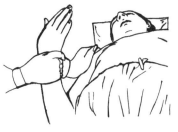

Figure 6. Testing elbow flexion.

Evidence Of Lower Motor Neuron (LMN) Weakness

Muscle wasting

Muscle wasting only occurs in lower motor neuron (LMN) type of weakness.

There is no muscle wasting in the upper motor neuron (UMN) type of weakness, unless it is long-standing, in which case it is due to disuse atrophy, e.g. calf wasting in stroke.

Loss of reflexes

Tendon jerks are lost in LMN type of weakness because motor part of the reflex arc is abolished.

Low tone

Lower motor neuron type weakness causes slackening of tone.
The limb is therefore easy to move as there is lower resistance because of lower tone.

6

What Causes LMN Weakness?

A. Damage to lower motor neurons which are:

1. Anterior horn cells in spinal cord, causing LMN weakness in the limbs, or cranial nerve nuclei in brainstem as in brainstem stroke, causing LMN cranial nerve palsies.

2. Nerve roots as in spinal nerve roots compressed by herniated discs, as in L5 root compression resulting in foot drop.

3. Peripheral nerves as in peripheral neuropathy.

4. Muscles as in myopathy.

Examples of LMN weakness

1. Quadriceps wasting in L3-L4 root compression.

As knee reflex is supplied by L3-L4 roots, the knee jerk is abolished.

2. Calf wasting in S1 root compression.

As ankle reflex is supplied by S1 root, therefore ankle jerk is lost. Other evidence of S1 root compression is also present, like sensory loss in the S1 distribution (lateral border of foot, little toe and over Achilles tendon).

3. Biceps wasting in C5/6 root compression.

    – Biceps jerk is supplied by C5/6 roots
    – Biceps jerk is therefore absent

This may form part of an interesting picture where biceps jerk is absent but triceps jerk is exaggerated due to cord compression at the same level, i.e. C5-C6.

Exaggerated triceps jerk is a UMN sign which is caused by compression of motor tracts in the cord at C5-6 level.

This is an example of a **mixed UMN/LMN picture.** Remember the level of the lesion is always at the level of LMN weakness, in this case C5-6. As compression is not selective and might impinge upon the cord, it would also cause UMN signs below the lesion by compressing the motor tracts.

What causes UMN weakness?

This is caused by damage to:

- Corticospinal fibres in the spinal cord, as in cord compression or spinal stroke.

- Pyramidal fibres in brainstem, as in brainstem stroke.

- Motor fibres in corona radiata, as in hemispheric stroke.

- Motor fibres in internal capsule, as in capsular stroke.

- Motor area in cerebral cortex, as in cortical stroke.

In a nutshell

LMN is: Anterior horn cells and below, namely: nerve roots, peripheral nerves and muscles.

UMN is: Cerebral cortex, corona radiata, internal capsule, corticobulbar, and corticospinal fibres.

What Are Fasciculations?

They are usually indicative of **dying neurons.**

You will see them whenever there is **LMN damage.**

By far the commonest cause is Motor Neuron Disease **(MND).**

In addition, calf muscle fasciculations may be seen in S1 root compression in spinal disc herniation (sciatica). They are also sometimes seen in the elderly, at times without any handy explanation.

Therefore, don't jump to MND unless other evidence is present.

Other evidence of MND includes atrophy of small hand muscles.

In MND you will also see **UMN signs** like increased tone in lower limbs, or exaggerated knee and ankle jerks.

MND can also cause **LMN wasting** and fasciculations in tongue, and palatal palsy causing dysphagia and dysarthria.

8

Tendon Jerks

Obtaining tendon jerks is an art like the golf swing. You can't learn it from a book. You simply need to practise.

Firstly learn how to swing the hammer.

1. **Never use the fancy paediatric** hammer kept on the trolley. Use the robust common rubber wheel on a flexible stick.

2. **Use your own flexor muscle** groups to hit the tendon. If you are driving a nail into the wall you don't hit it with a backward motion of your wrist!

3. **Position the limb before starting to test.**

For Upper Limbs

Place them in a flexed position resting partly on the patient's chest. Your left hand should be supporting each arm under the elbow in turn.

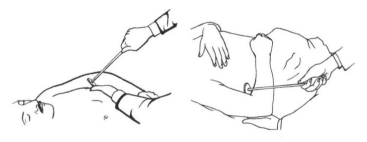

Figure 7. Left biceps jerk.   Figure 8. Right biceps jerk.

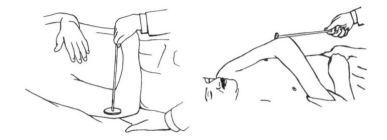

Figure 9. Right triceps jerk.   Figure 10. Left triceps jerk.

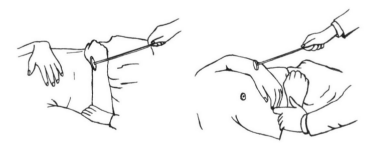

Figure 11. Right supinator jerk.   Figure 12. Left supinator jerk.

For Lower Limbs

Flex the knees with heels gently lying on the bed (not dug in). For ankles, flex the knee with the leg lying on its side (like a frog on its back, if both sides are tested together).

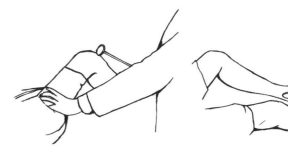

Figure 13. Testing knee jerk
(observe the quadriceps).

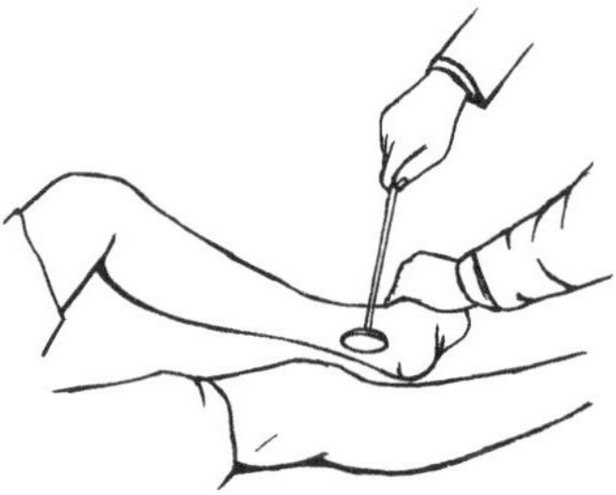

Figure 14. Testing ankle jerk
(observe the calf).

11

If Tendon Jerks Are Depressed Or Absent

It may be:

- **Lower motor neuron** weakness (then tone will also be decreased).

- Or you did not **use reinforcement**.

- Or **tone is so high** and limb so spastic that you can't get a jerk.

If this happens, try and elicit ankle clonus or patellar clonus.

Remember that you can get clonus with a hammer just like the tendon jerk. In fact while testing ankle jerks, you may get ankle clonus.

Plantars

They are often erroneously used as the sole neurological examination. This is like using pulse rate as the sole cardiac examination.

Any fault in technique can result in faulty result, colouring your diagnosis.

Golden Rule:

Never use plantars as your sole test to declare a lesion as UMN lesion.

How to get an extensor plantar response without really trying!

It is quite easy to get an extensor plantar response if you use the incorrect technique.

For instance, by taking the stimulus too far on the sole of the foot, or impinging on to the base of the big toe, you can produce extensor plantars in a normal patient.

Plantar Responses: Rules of Engagement

Rule Number One:

Never use plantars as your sole test to confirm a lesion as a UMN lesion.

Rule Number Two:

Use plantars only to support your suspicion of a UMN lesion, for instance, in conjunction with weakness and increased tone. (The exception to this rule is reduced tone and extensor plantars in Subacute Combined Degeneration of the Cord).

Alternative techniques to test plantars

You can also test for plantars by applying the stimulus underneath the lateral malleolus and curving round it anteriorly;

or applying pressure on to the shin with your thumb and index finger and moving them downwards.

Hemiplegic Gait

"It was as if I was tripping on matchsticks."

Comment by the patient who had stroke but did not know.

> **Q.** Hemiplegia causes UMN foot drop and foot drag. Why?
>
> **A.** Patient can't clear the ground as he can't lift his foot because spasticity keeps his knee stiff, preventing it from bending.

Result: Foot is dragged along instead of lifted.

14

Steppage Gait

"I had a spring in my step!"

(PG Wodehouse hero Bertie Wooster on getting out of a difficult love entanglement).

> **Q.** LMN weakness causes steppage gait. Why?
>
> **A.** A patient with LMN foot drop is able to lift his weak foot high enough to clear the ground as he is able to bend the knee (because there is no spasticity). LMN foot drop is a floppy foot and can only be cleared off the ground by raising the leg (steppage).

You can even **hear the steppage gait** through the flip flop noise if the patient is wearing slippers!

By contrast, a patient with UMN foot drop can't clear the ground because of spasticity. Therefore he has to drag his foot, thus producing the hemiplegic gait.

Parkinsonism

"Her feet were leaden with weights"

(About the heroine of a sad love story written by a famous female novelist).

In Parkinsonism there are two typical features

Firstly:

- Patient's feet appear to be stuck to the ground.

Secondly:

- There is slowness of movement (bradykinesia).

Three simple tricks to elicit bradykinesia

1. **Stare at the patient** and see who blinks first. If you blink first, the patient wins, but he probably has Parkinsonism!

2. Ask the patient to **get up and walk**. He takes a long time to get out of his chair, and a long time to start (start hesitation) and freezes in mid-stride.

3. Place a **chair next to the bed** and see if he can manoeuvre through the

narrow gap. If there is difficulty, think of Parkinsonism.

Tricks for confirming Parkinsonism

1. Look for rigidity and cog-wheeling at wrists.

2. Tremor, if seen, would be present at rest. If the tremor is of outstretched hands, it is action tremor (not Parkinsonism).

3. If tremor is not obvious, it can be accentuated by a simple trick.

4. Ask the patient to hit one knee with his hand alternately with the palm and the back of his hand. At the same time observe the other hand that is resting on his opposite knee, for any sign of a rest tremor.

5. Repeat the procedure on the other side.

Speech & Language

"Men of few words are the best men!" (Shakespeare)

Best use the term "aphasia" rather than "dysphasia" which unfortunately often gets written in the notes as "dysphagia"!

Receptive aphasia

The commonest mistake is to miss receptive aphasia as it is fluent. We think it is the patient's accent or the patient is presumed to be confused which is a very common and unfounded assumption with elderly patients.

Receptive aphasia is fluent aphasia

Golden Rule:

In a "confused" patient in a Stroke ward think of Receptive aphasia.

Patient's speech is fluent but he does not understand what he is saying and hence cannot correct himself. That is why it is called fluent. Often missed because the patient appears to be talking gibberish and therefore presumed to be confused!

Early receptive aphasia is even more difficult

You really have to listen to the patient very carefully for any slip ups.

Slip ups in patient's speech that should ring warning bells

Slip up No. 1: Phonemic paraphasia:

Examples: "pife" instead of "knife", "bar" instead of "car", "ben" instead of "pen".

Slip up No. 2: Verbal paraphasia:

Patient cannot name things but knows what you do with them. For instance, when you show him the object, "knife" is "something you cut with", "pen" is "something you write with".

Slip up No. 3: Another form:

In yet another form of **verbal paraphasia** the patient **will use an alternative word** like "car" for "van".

Three stages of receptive aphasia

You will notice 3 stages of receptive aphasia when you listen carefully to the patient.

1. Neologism:

New words that you have never heard before! Certainly not found in the Oxford dictionary!

2. Word salad:

In the next stage, the patient uses new words intermixed with known words so much so that it sounds like a word salad. Now the speech is full of words that you have never heard before.

3. Jargon aphasia:

Eventually speech becomes unintelligible although the patient is happily talking away without realizing there is anything wrong.

Patient is not upset or unhappy because he does not realize there is anything wrong.

Expressive aphasia

Speech is hesitant and becomes "telegraphic". Patient realizes there is a problem and becomes quite frustrated.

Example of Normal speech

"I will arrive by 10 PM train at King's Cross station tomorrow night. Please meet me outside the station's main entrance".

Before the advent of long distance phone calls and fax, and currently text messaging and emails, people used telegrams to communicate with each other as it was much quicker than sending a letter. However, it was prudent to use as few words as possible, in order to make it economical.

Therefore to save money we would condense the message in the form of a telegram, missing prepositions etc.

Converted into a Telegram

"Arrive King's Cross tomorrow meet outside".

The aphasic patient uses very few words, not to save money but because he has difficulty in findings words, i.e. he has limited vocabulary. He is therefore sending us a telegram!

Compare it with receptive aphasia where the patient finds words easily but they are gobbledegook.

Global Aphasia

If receptive and expressive aphasia occur together, it is called **global aphasia.** In severe forms the patient is **mute.**

The mysterious case of the globally aphasic Italian patient

Once the author saw an **Italian patient who did not speak any English but nobody knew that he didn't!**

Naturally he was diagnosed with global aphasia, as he had word finding difficulty in English (expressive component).

Moreover, he could not comprehend what was said to him **(receptive component).**

The author naturally greeted him with "buongiorno!" (part of his limited repertoire of Italian language).

The result was a torrent of Italian language by the beaming Italian. He was no longer aphasic!

17

Cerebellar Dysfunction

> **Q.** What is the major cause of toxic confusion in the physician?
>
> **A.** Cerebellar dysfunction

There are innumerable examples of a label of cerebellar ataxia where the patient had hemiparesis. Most of us can never get our heads round the difference. One even hears terms like "ataxia due to weakness".

> **Q.** How can you tell whether clumsiness during finger-nose test is cerebellar or due to paresis?
>
> **A.** Remember any weakness due to stroke will cause clumsiness in finger nose test. Therefore look at the whole picture. If there is weakness, it is not cerebellar

Golden Rule:

1. Never attempt to test cerebellar function in the presence of weakness. Any "clumsiness" due to weakness is just that. It is not ataxia.

2. Never label a tremor as cerebellar tremor, unless it is terminal intention tremor. Most likely it will turn out to be familial essential tremor. Ask about a parent with similar tremor at a similar age.

3. Never diagnose titubation as cerebellar for the same reason. Titubation and tremulous voice are also at components of Familial Essential Tremor, at times seen on their own.

A note of caution about cerebellar tremor

Remember this is terminal and occurs at the end of the excursion of the finger in the finger-nose test and that is why it is called terminal intention tremor (TIT).

Tricks to test cerebellar function

First make sure there is no weakness;

1. Then ask the patient to alternately **touch your finger and his nose.** Past pointing and TIT are present only if the patient has cerebellar dysfunction.

2. Ask patient to **tap back of one hand** with the palm of the other quickly. The affected hand is slow and clumsy. (This can happen in UMN weakness caused by stroke also, so make sure no weakness!).

3. **Heel-shin test.** Again make sure there is no weakness of either leg.

4. **Pendular knee jerks.** Make the patient sit on the edge of the bed and elevate the bed so that the patient's feet are dangling well above the ground. Normally a knee jerk has one prominent back and forth excursion. If the leg keeps going back and forth, back and forth, it is a pendular jerk. This can be used as a confirmatory test for cerebellar dysfunction.

Golden Rule:

1. Make sure that, while doing finger-nose test, **the upper arm is well away from the body.** If upper arm is adducted and supported (like resting on the bed) the patient can control the intention tremor.

2. Make sure that the tapping hand is raised 3 – 4 inches above the hand being tapped or the patient will be able to control the dysdiadokokinesia.

3. Again, make doubly sure that there is no weakness. Quite often there may appear to be cerebellar deficit because of weakness.

In fact, in a patient with anterior circulation stroke, a clumsy finger-nose test should be taken as a confirmation of hemiparesis, particularly when you find facial and leg weakness on the same side.

18

A Word About Nystagmus

We all get excited about nystagmus. Once seen, hey presto! "Cerebellar"! We forget that **nystagmus may be caused by vestibular damage** as well.

It can be evoked through tests like Hall Pike Manoeuvre for vestibular function as in BPPV (Benign Paroxysmal Positional Vertigo). So do not base your diagnosis solely on the presence of nystagmus.

A word about ataxia

Cerebellar ataxia is accentuated by asking the patient to do **tandem walk,** i.e. heel to toe walk. Remember to stay next to the patient to offer support in a patient with ataxia.

Do not confuse cerebellar ataxia with sensory ataxia which is caused by damage to posterior columns. This is best demonstrated through **Romberg's sign,** i.e. exaggerated swaying on closing eyes while standing. You will see positive Romberg's sign in Sub-acute Combined Degeneration of the Cord.

Simple trick to localize the lesion in cerebellar ataxia

Limb ataxia usually means damage to cerebellar hemispheres.

Truncal ataxia results from midline damage, e.g. vermis.

19

Eyes: Windows To The Diagnosis

Bilateral ptosis

This will be accompanied by evidence of frontalis action, i.e. wrinkling of forehead on attempting to look up. If there is no wrinkling of forehead on attempting to look up, it is an indication of myopathy. Ptosis in myasthenia is related to fatigue and will recover after rest.

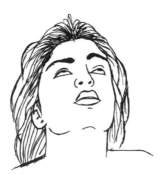

Figure 15. Bilateral ptosis with no frontalis action.

Ptosis in one eye

Unilateral ptosis is always due to 3rd nerve palsy (unless it is due to previous trauma or surgery). In a case with unilateral ptosis, don't forget to look for a "down and out eye".

Horner's syndrome is not a true ptosis as the patient can open the affected eye fully if asked to do so.

I spy with my little eye something beginning with H!

- In **Horner's syndrome,** the eye appears small and the pupil is also small.

- This is opposite of fight or flight.

- The reason is cervical sympathetic paralysis.

- The eye appears small because palpebral fissure is narrowed. The eye has a sunken appearance but there is no true ptosis.

- The voluntary control is retained and ptosis will disappear if patient is asked to look up.

- In a dark room the normal pupil will dilate but the abnormal pupil will remain small.

- You will also find loss of sweating on the same side of face. The ptosis in Horner's Syndrome is pseudo-ptosis.

Another example of pseudo-ptosis

Sometimes the patient keeps the affected eye shut in 6th nerve palsy, in order to avoid troublesome diplopia.

Note that the eye is shut or nearly shut in 3rd nerve palsy anyway (true ptosis).

In pseudo-ptosis, either due to Horner's Syndrome or patient's attempt to avoid diplopia, the patient will open his affected eye fully when asked to do so.

Pupils & The Light Pathway

Q.   Light shone into one eye constricts both pupils. Why?

A.

1.   The light from one eye passes in **optic nerve** fibres on to the **superior colliculus** in the midbrain on the same side.

2.   Each superior colliculus receives fibres from both sides because of crossing of optic tracts.

3.   Fibres from superior colliculus then connect, via **pretectal area** of the midbrain, to **Edinger Westphal** nuclei on both sides.

4.   These are the parasympathetic fibres which travel via the **ciliary ganglion** on each side and connect to **constrictor pupillae** muscles of the iris on each side.

This is the basis for direct and consensual reflex. It is thus obvious that both pupils will react simultaneously when light is shone into either eye.

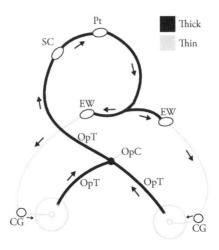

Figure 16. Light pathway.

Thick arrows: Afferent pathway from Optic Nerve.

Thin arrows: Efferent or parasympathetic supply to constrictor pupillae muscles.

Op T = Optic Tract Op C = Optic Chiasma S C = Superior Colliculus Pt = Pretectal Area

E W = Edinger Westphal Nucleus

C G = Ciliary Ganglion

Ptosis with un-dilated pupil

If you find a **3rd nerve lesion** (ptosis and abducted eye) **but pupil is not dilated,** then it is due to 3rd nerve infarction.

The parasympathetic fibres from Edinger Westphal nucleus which constrict the pupil are located on the periphery of the third nerve fascicle. They will get damaged by compression from outside, e.g. by an aneurysm of posterior communicating artery. This will cause dilatation of the pupil along with ptosis and eye turned down and out **(surgical 3rd nerve palsy).**

However, infarction of 3rd nerve causes deeper damage, thus sparing the constrictor fibres (which are located on the outside).

The pupil is therefore of normal size but there is ptosis and eye is moved down and out **(medical 3rd nerve palsy).** Commonest cause is Type II Diabetes Mellitus.

Dilated pupil in an unconscious patient

This is a medical emergency

Unilateral or bilateral ptosis with dilated pupil on one or both sides means:

Temporal lobe herniation or coning which is dragging or stretching the 3rd nerve.

The patient should be transferred to ICU straightaway. Management must not be delayed even to wait for a CT scan. Once both pupils are dilated, chances of recovery are remote.

Dilated pupil in a conscious patient

1. Posterior communicating artery aneurysm compressing or stretching the ipsilateral 3rd nerve.

2. Weber's Syndrome (midbrain infarction) with ipsilateral 3rd nerve palsy and contralateral hemiparesis (crossed palsy).

3. Mydriasis from an earlier fundoscopy often performed in A&E (always ask about eye drops).

What is Marcus Gunn Pupil?

Observe the magical light that dilates the pupil instead of constricting it!

In unilateral optic atrophy, the afferent or sensory pathway is damaged due to atrophy. Light shone into the affected pupil cannot constrict either ipsilateral (direct reflex) or contralateral pupil (through consensual reflex) because the message is not getting through.

However, when you shine the light into the normal pupil, both pupils will react because the message is passing through the normal side to both eyes.

Now when you bring back the light quickly to the affected pupil, it is hitting the damaged afferent fibres again. The affected pupil which had previously constricted consensually (i.e. it had worked through the normal side), will now appear to dilate!

You can rapidly move the light from one eye to the other to view the strange spectacle of light dilating the affected pupil instead of constricting it!

This is called **Swinging Light Reflex.** The affected pupil is called **Marcus Gunn Pupil.**

Diplopia

False image is always lateral. Block the affected eye and it will go away. The patient learns to do that himself.

Check which eye. Test 6th and 3rd nerves.

Trick to remember

If you find a 6th Nerve palsy, always remember to look for an LMN facial palsy.

This combination indicates a pontine stroke.

In the below diagram, false image is to the patient's left (i.e. at the end of the broken line) while the true image is to the right of the false image (i.e., at the end of converging solid lines).

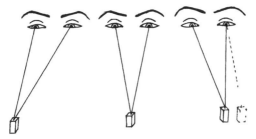

Figure 17. Diplopia to the left.

21

Why Are 6th And 7th Nerves Sometimes Involved Together?

In pons, the 7th nerve fascicle wraps round 6th nerve nucleus. So they both get involved together in pontine infarction.

There is also contralateral UMN hemiparesis indicative of crossed palsy seen in brainstem strokes.

Golden Rule:

Eye not abducting: 6th Nerve
Eye not adducting: 3rd Nerve

Remember the 6th nerve nucleus is located in pons and the 3rd nerve nucleus in the midbrain.

What can the car steering wheel teach us about eyes?

Medial Longitudinal Fasciculus works in the same way as a pinion and rack mechanism in the car steering. It makes the two wheels (eyes) move in unison in either direction.

It connects the 3rd Nerve nucleus in midbrain to the opposite 6th Nerve nucleus in pons.

If it is damaged, on moving the steering to the left (i.e. when the patient attempts to **look to the left), the left wheel (eye) moves fully but judders** (has nystagmus) and the right wheel (eye) only moves half way. The same will happen when you move the steering (eyes) to the right. This is known as **posterior internuclear opthalmoplegia or "one and a half syndrome".**

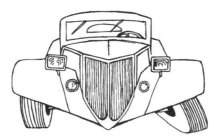

Figure 18. Left wheel is out of alignment due to axle break and judders on moving the steering to left while right wheel only moves half way.

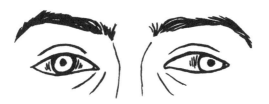

Figure 19. Posterior Internuclear opthalmoplegia (one and a half syndrome).

In this situation, with the patient trying to look left, the right eye is only moving halfway, while the left eye moves all the way but is juddering, i.e. shows nystagmus.

In the same patient, when he attempts to look right, the left eye goes only half way, while the right eye goes all the way but judders (has nystagmus).
If the steering mechanism is completely broken down, both wheels of the car are turned outwards, making any steering impossible.

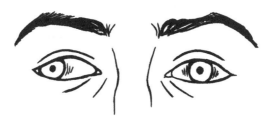

Figure 20. Posterior internuclear opthalmoplegia (one and a half syndrome). With the patient trying to look right, the left eye is only moving halfway while right eye shows juddering (nystagmus).

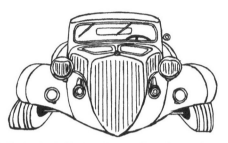

Figure 21. Both wheels "looking" outwards with complete axle break.

In a patient with this problem, both eyes would be looking outwards. This is known as **WEBINO** (Wall eyed bilateral internuclear opthalmoplegia).

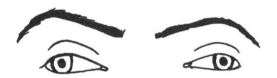

22

Midbrain Infarction

Weber's Syndrome

Ipsilateral

3rd Nerve palsy (dilated pupil which is down and out).

Contralateral

Upper Motor Neuron weakness on opposite side. This is called "crossed palsy", meaning cranial nerve on the same side (LMN) and arm and leg weakness on the opposite side (UMN).

A cranial nerve nucleus is LMN, like anterior horn cells in spinal cord.

The contralateral hemiparesis is always UMN like in a cortical stroke.

Benedikt's Syndrome

Ipsilateral: 3rd Nerve palsy
Contralateral: Ataxia

Ataxia is caused by infarction of red nucleus which has connections to opposite cerebellum.

Nothnagel's Syndrome

Ipsilateral: 3rd Nerve palsy
Also ipsilateral: Ataxia (superior cerebellar peduncle)

23

Pontine Infarction

Ipsilateral: 6th and 7th nerve palsies

This is because 7th nerve fascicle wraps round 6th nucleus and also the nerves exit together.

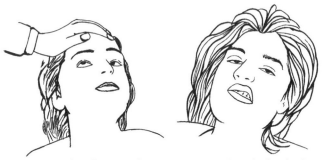

Figure 23. Right 6th nerve palsy in pontine stroke.

Figure 24. Right facial palsy in pontine stroke.

Note that the right eye is deviated medially (right Lateral Rectus Palsy).
In the same patient, you can see LMN weakness of right side of face.

Plus contralateral UMN hemiplegia just like in a "normal" case of hemiplegic stroke.

Remember the 6th and 7th nerve palsies in pontine infarction are LMN. Therefore facial weakness will be like Bell's palsy.

This can be missed if you concentrate only on hemiparesis. Or you might concentrate only on facial palsy and miss the stroke altogether, confusing it with Bell's palsy!

Golden Rule:

In a case of LMN facial palsy:

- Always test eye movements to see if facial weakness is accompanied by lateral rectus palsy (inability to abduct the eye) on the same side.

- This gives us an idea whether lesion is in pons.

- Also test opposite side for any UMN weakness in arm or leg. Why?

A: Because a brainstem stroke causes crossed palsy (ipsilateral cranial nerve and contralateral UMN weakness).

24

Medullary Infarction

(Lateral Medullary Syndrome or Wallenberg Syndrome)

Ipsilateral findings:

- Facial sensory loss (Trigeminal fibres)

- Horner's Syndrome (cervical sympathetics)

- Ataxia (inferior cerebellar peduncle)

- Hoarseness and dysphagia (9th and 10th nerve nuclei)

Contralateral findings:

- Hemi-sensory loss (spinothalamic fibres), because sensory fibres having crossed lower down (crossing of spinothalamic tracts), sensory loss is on the opposite side.

25

Facial Weakness

Facial weakness in stroke is almost always UMN type. So much so that we forget that stroke can cause LMN facial weakness as well, like in pontine stroke where it is on the same side as the infarct, with UMN weakness of arm and leg on the opposite side (crossed palsy).

In midbrain and pons, motor fibres have not crossed as yet, so if there is an infarct, the opposite side gets UMN weakness (like in a hemispheric stroke).

However, because cranial nerve nuclei that are also involved, are located on the same side, you get signs of cranial nerve damage **on the same side.**
Therefore, in pontine stroke, you get **6th and 7th weakness on the same side plus UMN palsy of the opposite half of the body.**

This is called **Millard Gubler Syndrome,** which is a good example of crossed palsy. In this you will see weakness of eye abduction causing diplopia on the same side and also facial palsy on the same side. Don't forget contralateral hemiparesis.

26

Tremor

Golden Rule:

1. Never diagnose tremor as cerebellar unless you have done detailed neurology.

2. Never diagnose Parkinsonism on the basis of tremor alone. Always look for bradykinesia.

Action Tremor

Any tremor of outstretched arms is an action tremor as opposed to rest tremor. "Physiological" tremor in thyrotoxicosis is an action tremor. Cerebellar tremor is also an action tremor.

Cerebellar tremor or terminal intention tremor

This is in fact an action tremor with something extra, i.e. it is a terminal intention tremor, which means the tremor is most intense when the finger reaches its mark. It is accompanied by past pointing, which means the finger keeps going off the mark, either to one side or the other.

What does titubation have to do with cerebellar tremor?

Answer: Very little

Benign Familial or Benign Essential tremor

Is the commonest action tremor. It is sometimes accompanied by titubation and tremor of the voice, which have the same mechanism.

It is frequently and mistakenly diagnosed as a "cerebellar tremor" or even Parkinsonism.

Do not use these labels unless you have examined the patient for other evidence of cerebellar dysfunction or Parkinsonism.

Dystonic tremor

Observe the patient "wrestling" with himself

- You might have seen arm wrestling in movies.

- Our diehard cop hero and the bad guy straining so hard against each other that their arms seem to be shaking with effort.

- This is the same as dystonic tremor.

- In normal movement when you want to use one muscle group, the opposing muscle group automatically relaxes.

- In dystonia both the opposing muscle groups remain active. The result is either an attitude of contortion depending on which muscle group wins, or a constant jerky movement as in **Spasmodic torticollis, or Writer's cramp.**

- **The opposing muscle groups are working simultaneously** and so hard that the limb or the neck is shaking and straining with the effort **as if the patient is wrestling with himself!**

- The commonest example of dystonia is spasmodic torticollis.

Rest tremor

If you see tremor at rest be sure to assess the patient for Parkinsonism as follows:

1. Observe the face for reduced blinking (evidence of bradykinesia).

2. If **the patient can win the staring match** against you he may have Parkinsonism.

3. Ask the patient to **play the piano** with outstretched arms and see if there is clumsiness due to bradykinesia.

4. Remember clumsiness can also be due to hemiparesis but then there will be other evidence of hemiparesis.

5. Check for **cog-wheeling** at the wrists.

How to accentuate the rest tremor

Ask the patient to put both hands on his knees and strike each knee rapidly

with each hand alternately. Observe the other hand for any rest tremor.

27

Paraparesis And Finding The Level Of Lesion

Sensory level

When you suspect spinal cord compression, always check sensory level with a neuro-pin which is possibly the cheapest implement that is not even kept in some stroke units!

- T7/8 below rib margin
- T10 at umbilicus
- T12 at inguinal region

Weakness in cord compression

In cord compression, it is always a combination of UMN + LMN.

Golden Rule:

UMN below the lesion, LMN at the level of lesion.

To find the level of the lesion, look for the level at which you find LMN signs.

Scenario 1

High cervical compression

This patient was found to have exaggerated jerks in all the four limbs.

Q. What imaging mode is to be requested?

A. MRI cervical spine to rule out **high cord compression.**

Scenario 2

Mid-cervical compression

In this patient both lower limb jerks were exaggerated. This means the problem has to be **spinal** (unless there was a recent stroke plus a history of a previous stroke).

Exaggerated lower limb jerks on their own do not give us the level of the lesion.

However, if in the above patient you found an absence of biceps jerks, this should alert you to the Golden Rule which is "LMN at the site of the lesion". Biceps is supplied by C5-6. Therefore lesion is at C5-6. Exaggerated knee and ankle jerks is a UMN sign which does not give us a clue about the level of the lesion.

You might also find exaggerated triceps jerks (C7) in this patient. This is a UMN sign too and confirms the principle:
"UMN Below The Lesion"

Trick to remember:

Lower limb jerks are always exaggerated in cord compression at any level. They are supplied by L3-4, (knee jerk) and S1 (ankle jerk) which is well below any site of cord compression.

That Golden Rule again

"LMN at the level of the lesion; UMN below the lesion."

Scenario 3

Compression at mid-thoracic level

- Intercostal and abdominal muscles weakened but difficult to test (LMN).

- Both lower limb jerks exaggerated (UMN).

Q. What imaging mode would you request?

A. MRI thoracic spine to rule out **mid-thoracic compression.**

Scenario 4

Compression at lumbosacral levels
Only nerve roots are involved because cord ends at L1-2

Some lower spinal root compressions:

L3-4:
* Absent knee jerk.

* Sensory loss medial aspect of thigh and lower leg and front of knee.

L5:
* Weakness of dorsiflexion causing foot drop.

* Sensory loss lateral aspect of leg and at dorsum of foot.

S1:
* Absent ankle jerk

* Sensory loss at lateral border of foot.

S3-4:
* Saddle anaesthesia and bladder involvement.

> **Q.** In one of the above situations what imaging would you request?
>
> **A.** MRI **lumbo-sacral spine.**

A note of caution

If you find absent or depressed tendon jerks in all the four limbs, always remember GBS (Guillain-Barre Syndrome) and involve a senior as this is a life threatening emergency on account of respiratory muscle involvement.

Magic formula for lower limb jerks

Q. Normal knee jerks + absent ankle jerks?

A. Peripheral Neuropathy

Q. Absent knee jerks + normal ankle jerks ?

A. Myopathy (as weakness in myopathy is almost always proximal)

28

Bladder Problems

With UMN lesion

As in stroke, intracranial space occupying lesion, hydrocephalus etc. UMN causes spasticity.

An easy way to remember this is to think of the bladder as also being "spastic".

What will happen?

There is loss of capacity and bladder tone is high with hyper-reflexia of bladder. As soon as bladder fills up a little bit, the patient wants to pass urine.

Result is Urgency incontinence.

With LMN lesion

There is loss of tone. Think of bladder also becoming "flaccid" in line with the nature of LMN lesion (low tone).

If the bladder becomes like a large flaccid balloon, it can hold a lot of urine so there will be urinary retention and absence of sensation of bladder fullness.

Result is large volume of urine in the bladder.

This causes overflow incontinence

The end result is the same as with an enlarged prostate which hinders the complete emptying of the bladder.

Warning:

Do not let dribbling of small amounts of urine fool you. This patient is not passing urine normally. A bladder scan will show residual urine.

Reflex or Automatic Bladder

- The bladder fills and empties automatically.

- Emptying may be accompanied by autonomic phenomenon like sweating.

- Emptying can be aided by stimulation of anal or scrotal skin.

These patients are often seen in Spinal Trauma Units and bladder problem accompanies paraparesis.

29

Presentations Mistaken For Stroke

- Weakness and wasting of **small hand muscles in C8-T1** root lesion (LMN lesion). Also known as claw hand. The usual cause is **cervical rib or band,** or Pancoast tumour. It may be accompanied by Horner's Syndrome due to compression of cervical sympathetics.

- Weakness of **quadriceps in L3-4 lesion.** Knee jerk on affected side is absent and not brisk, as it would be in a stroke. Why?

- A: L3-4 root compression causes.

- LMN weakness and therefore absent knee jerk.

- Weakness of shoulder abduction in **brachial plexus injury.** There is wasting of shoulder girdle muscles (C5 root) and upper limb is floppy with low tone.

- **Foot drop in L5 root** lesion but tone will be low as it is LMN lesion. (Contrast it with stroke where there is foot drop but tone is greatly increased at the ankle).

- **Bell's palsy** is by far the commonest presentation which is mistaken for stroke.

Common stroke mimics referred to A&E as stroke

- **Postictal** palsy
- **Functional** symptomatology
- **BPPV** (Benign Paroxysmal Positional Vertigo) is commonly mistaken for posterior circulation stroke or TIA and referred to the TIA clinic.
- **Migraine**
- Cerebral **tumour**
- **Previous stroke** (and worsening of weakness as a result of UTI in nursing home residents.).
- **Bell's palsy**

What is claw hand?

This results from the pull of long tendons in the absence of small hand muscles. There is imbalance of tension between long tendons and short intrinsic muscles. The stabilizing influence of small muscles is gone.
Site of lesion is C8/T1.

Common causes:

- **MND** (Motor Neuron Disease)
- **Pancoast** tumour causing C8/T1 root compression in the neck, accompanied by Horner's syndrome due to involvement of cervical sympathetics.
- **Syringomyelia**

The two "drops": wrist drop & foot drop

Wrist drop:

UMN: Stroke

LMN: Radial Nerve compression, e.g., in **"Saturday Night Palsy"** through pressure on Radial groove from the back of the chair while asleep usually under the influence of alcohol.

Foot drop:

UMN: Stroke

Gait in UMN foot drop: Foot drag. Patient can't lift his foot as he can't bend his knee due to spasticity.

LMN:

1.   L5 root compression in Lumbar disc herniation.

2.   Compression of Common Peroneal nerve at neck of fibula ("Crossed Leg Palsy").

Gait in LMN foot drop: High steppage gait as the patient is unable to clear the ground unless he lifts the leg to clear the dangling foot off the ground.

30

Functional Symptomatology

Important to remember:

A patient with functional symptomatology is **not malingering.**

- **Symptoms are genuine to the patient** and the result of subconscious mechanisms. However, the patient appears not to be too concerned.

- Patient is caught up in an intolerable situation. **Symptoms are a way out.**

Tests:

1. **Drop sign** – "Paralysed" hand falls away to the side if lifted and dropped on to the chest.

2. **Hoover's Sign** – "Paralysed" leg presses down on bed when resistance applied to elevation of normal leg.

3. **If Grade 4 weakness, it is jerky** when resistance is applied, as opposing muscle groups are working at the same time. It looks as if the patient is straining very hard and arm wrestling with himself.

4. **Adductor test** – With the patient lying in bed, "paralysed" leg adducts at the same time that the patient is asked to adduct normal leg while applying resistance to both the legs.

Functional Sensory Loss

- Well defined **boundaries with sharp edges** of sensory loss exactly in the midline. A rare exception to this rule is thalamic infarct where the sensory loss boundaries are well defined.

- **No sensory loss at the back.**

- **Intensity and boundaries keep changing from one examination to another.**

- Patient appears **unconcerned.**

Functional Fits

The patient **rarely hurts** himself. Usually manages to fall into a convenient chair or on to the bed.

- **Tongue biting is rare.**

- Patient may be conscious while having a generalised fit.

- Fits occur most commonly in front of an **audience** and therefore observed by family or nurses, or observed during consultant's ward round.

Trick to Remember: Functional fits may occur in a genuinely epileptic patient and interspersed with genuine fits.

How to tell whether a fit is genuine

- **History of tonic-clonic** phase followed by sleep. Patient wakes up confused and headachy.

- **Voiding urine** during fit.

- **Injury** during fit.

- Always look for a **tongue bite** usually on the side of the tongue.

- Ask if sometimes **wakes up with headache** or body pains (sign that patient had a fit in the night).

Golden Rule: Don't forget witness statements. Best investigation of a fit is collateral story.

When might a fit be functional?

- Always in the presence of **onlookers.**

- Patient usually doesn't get hurt.

- Results from intolerable home or work situation.

- Unlike malingering, patient is unaware.

- Patient is strangely unconcerned.

Mixed genuine and functional fits

- **Several kinds of fits,** mostly atypical.

- Fits were **previously under control.**

- Fits look generalised but patient mostly **conscious.**

Fit or syncope?

- In **vasovagal syncope** patient **comes round** the minute his head hits the ground.

- In syncope, patient goes **pale** and not blue.

- **Cardiac syncope can cause fit** due to cerebral anoxia.

EEG reports and physicians

EEG reports are successful attempts to obfuscate and confuse the reader. The report frequently does not contain the conclusion and keeps you guessing (neurologists often do this!).

How to make sense of an EEG Report

Look whether the report mentions:
- Slow waves or sharp waves.

Then look where they are located:
- Frontally, temporally or parietally.

Don't be overawed by terms like alpha, beta or theta activity which are only variations of normal rhythms.

Rules of thumb when looking at an EEG

1. Slow waves and sharp waves indicate epileptic discharges.

2. Temporal slow waves: HSE (Herpes Simplex Encephalitis).

3. Generalised slow waves: Encephalopathy.

4. Lots of spikes or sharp waves: Recent fit or uncontrolled epilepsy.

31

Headaches That Mystify

Tension Headache

- Long history with no physical effects.

- Might be present on getting up in the morning.

- Waxing and waning intensity but never seems to go off completely.

- Mainly located occipitally and in the neck but moves frontally.

Management

Keep analgesic drugs to the minimum. Try Amitriptyline at a dose of 25 mg nightly. Start with smaller dose of 10 mg.

Migraine

- **Aura** may be present and then usually visual.

- **Definite onset.**

- Photophobia, noise phobia, nausea, vomiting.

- Usually terminated by going to sleep.

- In older patients aura may not be followed by headache.

Migraine as a stroke mimic

Patients throng to the TIA clinic due to visual or sensory aura. In fact, due to increased awareness, **migraine has almost doubled the TIA patient load** in some hospitals. This is now bread and butter for the young and enthusiastic stroke physicians and a source of much intellectual conjecturing. However this does not mean that migraine cannot be associated with stroke or itself cause a stroke.

Tumour headache

- **Recent** onset.

- **Constant headache** with nausea and vomiting.

- Other physical effects like **weight loss.**

- There may be some **neurological deficit.**

Subarachnoid Haemorrhage

- Like a hammer blow or **thunderclap.**

- **Neck stiffness** and nausea or vomiting.

- Constant and does not subside like a migraine.

Analgesic Abuse Headache

- Initially presents as **migraine or tension** headache.

- History dating back to **months or years.**

- Usually shows characteristics of **tension headache.**

- **Never goes off completely.**

- Worsens as soon as the last dose of paracetamol wears off, until the patient takes another dose.

Management

- **Reassurance.** Do CT of the head to reassure.

- Stop analgesic, almost always Paracetamol, often used by the patient and physician indiscriminately.

- **Bed time Amitriptyline.**

32

3 Minutes Neurology In A Sitting Patient

1. Put hand on each thigh alternately and ask patient to lift leg with knee flexed: 10 seconds.

2. Put hand on dorsum of each foot alternately and apply resistance while patient tries to dorsiflex the foot: 10 seconds.

3. Do the same by applying resistance against plantar flexion alternately: 15 seconds.

4. Ask patient to lift both arms overhead and then back down to his sides, first without and then against resistance: 20 seconds.

5. Ask patient to "play piano" with outstretched arms: 10 seconds.

6. Ask patient to tap back of one hand with the palm of the other hand alternately: 10 seconds.

7. Do finger-nose test: 15 seconds.

8. Test grip of each hand by asking patient to squeeze your two fingers (never one). Or, in case of an obviously strong person, ask him to clench fist while you try to open it: 15 seconds.

9. Ask patient to flex and extend a clenched fist while you try to oppose it: 10 seconds.

10. Ask patient to flex and extend elbow while you hold the patient's wrist and apply resistance: 15 seconds.

11. Ask patient to show teeth and then screw eyes shut: 10 seconds.

12. Ask patient to open mouth, say "Ah" and stick tongue out to move it from side to side: 10 seconds.

13. Ask patient to follow your finger left, then right and at the same time ask whether he sees one finger or two: 10 seconds.

14. Block patient's one eye and test visual fields alternatively in all four quadrants: 20 seconds.

Total: 3 minutes

33

Revision

Examining the unconscious patient

Q. Head and eyes turned to one side in stroke. Why?

A. Normal cortex pushes head and eyes to the other side. That means the opposite cortex is not functioning.

For instance, head and eyes turned to left means:

Right hemisphere is the active hemisphere and left hemisphere is not functioning, which means right hemiparesis.

Fine Print

In a patient who is having an epileptic fit, head and eyes are turned to the side that is fitting. This is caused by the epileptic discharges on the contralateral side, which temporarily becomes the "active" side.

Limb Weakness

Q. How can you tell whether weakness is UMN or LMN type?

A. Increased tone means weakness is UMN type.
Decreased tone means weakness is LMN type.

Tendon Jerks

Use of hammer is an art, like a golf swing. Use your flexor groups. You don't hit a nail with a hammer with a backward movement of your wrist (wrist extension).

Exaggerated = UMN. You may get clonus.
Depressed = LMN. But always use reinforcement.

Gait

Q. What is the difference between foot drag, steppage and shuffling?

A. Foot drag is hemiparetic (i.e. UMN, so the patient can't bend knee to lift leg due to spasticity.

Steppage is due to the patient successfully clearing the ground as there is no spasticity. However, due to "floppy foot drop" the affected foot is raised unnaturally high, which is a conscious effort on the part of the patient to stop his dangling toes hitting the ground.

Shuffle is due to bradykinesia or slowing of movement as in Parkinsonism.

Speech

Q. Is unintelligible speech receptive or expressive aphasia?

A. Receptive aphasia

The speech is fluent but unintelligible because the patient is unable to correct himself as he can't follow his own speech (jargon aphasia). In a milder case, there are new words or neologism.

Expressive Aphasia means word finding difficulty, so there are fewer words. The patient stops and starts trying to find a word, often unsuccessfully and frustratingly shaking his head.

Cerebellar function

Q. Can you have ataxia and weakness in the same patient?

A. Do not test cerebellar function in the presence of weakness.

The weakness indicates that the patient has hemiparesis. The "ataxia" or clumsiness in a patient with hemiparesis is due to weakness and not due to cerebellar dysfunction.

Q. Is tremor a sign of cerebellar dysfunction if the patient can't do finger-nose test?

A. Only a tremor that is terminal intention tremor and accompanied by past pointing is cerebellar. Mere clumsiness may be due to paresis. Then one must look for other evidence of hemiparesis.

Q. Is nystagmus a conclusive evidence of cerebellar dysfunction?

A. Nystagmus may be vestibular, so you must check for other evidence of cerebellar dysfunction before committing yourself.

Ptosis in one eye

Caused by 3rd nerve lesion, so also look for dilated pupil and down and out eye. If 3rd nerve lesion is obvious, as the eye is down and out, but the pupil is not dilated, think of 3rd nerve infarction, which can happen in a diabetic patient.

> **Q.** What is the difference between ptosis in 3rd nerve palsy and Horner's syndrome?
>
> **A.** If unilateral ptosis, but small pupil, think of Horner's Syndrome. Patient is able to open eye fully when asked to do so.

Warning: Unilateral "ptosis" may actually be voluntary (pseudo-ptosis), which is an attempt to avoid diplopia.

Unilateral Dilated Pupil

> **Q.** Is a unilateral dilated pupil a sign of impending disaster?
>
> **A.** Unless there is evidence that the pupil was dilated earlier with mydriatics, you must take it seriously. You must ask the A&E staff whether somebody had put mydriatics in the eye.

If patient conscious:

Posterior communicating artery aneurysm. There has been a leakage inside the aneurysm wall, which becomes bigger and compresses the 3rd Nerve.

If patient unconscious:

Coning or temporal lobe herniation stretching the 3rd Nerve. Very serious situation. Chances of recovery are nil once both pupils dilate. Patient is deeply comatose.

Diplopia

False image always lateral.

> **Q.** If eye adducted, also look for ipsilateral LMN facial weakness and contralateral hemiparesis. Why?
>
> **A.** 6th and 7th nerves are located very close together in pons and pontine infarction will involve both.

Parkinsonism

> **Q.** If suspected, try to outstare patient. Why?
>
> **A.** Reduced blinking is a prominent early feature of facial bradykinesia before the patient develops mask-like face.

"This guide to neurological examination aims to make these clinical skills more accessible and less mysterious to medical students and junior doctors. It succeeds in doing this by clarity, prioritising the common pitfalls and not a little humour. It is a valuable adjunct to the more weightier tomes".

Dr. Phil Earnshaw, Clinical Tutor and PACES Examiner, University Hospital of North Durham.

"This book helps to demystify my murky understanding of neurology from medical school. It has clear concise tips which are useful in a practical sense. Would have been very useful if given at the start of, or during, a medical school neurology attachment!   Favourite parts are 3 minute neurology examination and the golden rules".

Dr. Francis Campbell, GP trainee, Great Western Hospital, Swindon.

"This book is the cream of a neurologist's experience presented to students in a way that makes neurology easier to master."

Dr. Rafik Henry, Consultant Stroke Physician, Good Hope Hospital, Sutton Coldfield.

"I feel confident in doing neurological examination now. The 3 minute neurological examination will make it easier for all junior doctors to assess the CNS."

Dr. Sobia Hina, SHO in Elderly Medicine.

"Very easy to read. I like the easy ways to remember things. The examples are really useful. I like the how to examine section".

Dr. Jenny Millard, F2. Department of Stroke Medicine, Great Western Hospital, Swindon.

"Good to repeat things and I like the questions throughout and the end of the book quiz. Some diagrams may be a good idea".

Dr. Rachel Campbell, GP trainee, Swindon.

"Straight to the point. Easy to follow for the junior doctors".

Dr. Marek Kunc, Consultant Neurologist, Airedale Hospital, Yorkshire.

"I should congratulate Dr Khawaja for use of such simple language making it easy for any reader to understand neurological terms. I also liked the humour that he has used which has made the reading enjoyable, something you would normally not expect in reading of Neurology which is usually perceived as a dry subject especially among junior doctors. Use of schematic drawings which he is planning to do would certainly add up to the flavour."

Dr. Mahesh Dhakal, Consultant Stroke Physician, University Hospital of North Durham.

"Congratulations on writing such a concise and easy to follow booklet.
I know the main focus is on neurological examination, but the two common acute presentations which are acute onset headache and fits, if they can be incorporated, would complete the work and cover most of it for junior doctors."

Dr. M. Safeer Abbasi, Consultant Physician, Clinical Tutor and PACES Examiner Pinderfield Hospital, Wakefield.

"This booklet is thoughtful and practical in guiding clinicians through an often difficult set of neurological presentations."

Dr. Jon Miles, Consultant Chest Physician and Clinical Director in Medicine, Rotherham General Hospital.

Lightning Source UK Ltd.
Milton Keynes UK
UKOW06f0225221215

265157UK00001B/1/P